Distribution, publication, and copying in any form are prohibited and subject to damages.

TEN HYPNOSES

Copying, publishing, and sharing with third parties are only permitted with the written consent of the author. Please observe the notes on copyright and usage.

Distribution, publication, and copying in any form are prohibited and subject to damages.

Copying, publishing, and sharing with third parties are only permitted with the written consent of the author. Please observe the notes on copyright and usage.

Distribution, publication, and copying in any form are prohibited and subject to damages.

Ingo Michael Simon

TEN HYPNOSES

4

REDUCING OVERWEIGHT, SLIMMING DOWN

Copying, publishing, and sharing with third parties are only permitted with the written consent of the author. Please observe the notes on copyright and usage.

Distribution, publication, and copying in any form are prohibited and subject to damages.

© 2024 Ingo Michael Simon
All rights reserved.
Independently published
www.ingosimon.com

Important Notes for Urgent Attention:
The contents of this book are based on the practical experiences of the author with hypnosis applications and psychotherapy in a trance state. Although the author has strived for the utmost care, errors or misunderstandings in the presentation cannot be completely excluded. Therapeutic work with people and the application of hypnosis are solely the responsibility of the hypnotist. It cannot be ruled out that parts of this book may be misunderstood or that the application of a presented procedure may cause an undesirable reaction in the client. The author also assumes no co-responsibility if work with a client is carried out with reference to the statements in this book.

The Author:
Ingo Michael Simon studied psychology and education and is a hypnotherapist with practices in southwestern Germany and Switzerland. With the help of hypnosis-supported psychotherapy, he primarily treats people with persistent psychological conditions. His practice focuses on anxiety disorders, pathological compulsions, and psychosomatic illnesses. His therapeutic offerings mainly include classical and modern hypnosis applications and the dreamland therapy he developed himself.

Copying, publishing, and sharing with third parties are only permitted with the written consent of the author. Please observe the notes on copyright and usage.

Notes on Copyright and Usage

Copying, publishing, and sharing with third parties is prohibited and only permitted with the written consent of the author. Please observe the following copyright and usage guidelines.

This work has been carefully crafted and created to the best of the author's knowledge and personal experience. It comprises text templates and application guidelines for professional hypnosis sessions. The author is a licensed psychotherapist with extensive experience in psychotherapy, coaching, and personal training using hypnotic techniques and methods. Nevertheless, the author and the publisher assume no liability for the accuracy of information, instructions, and advice, nor for any typographical errors. The author and publisher accept no responsibility or liability for the application of these texts and recommendations with clients or patients, nor for any potential consequences or unexpected reactions. It is expressly noted that the application of therapeutic and advisory techniques and formulations lies solely and entirely within the responsibility of the practitioner. This also applies to adherence to the boundaries of legally regulated medical and therapeutic practices. The fact that a book containing action proposals is freely available for sale does not imply that its application with clients or patients is permitted for everyone.

Distribution, publication, and copying in any form are prohibited and subject to damages.

Copying, publishing, and sharing with third parties are only permitted with the written consent of the author. Please observe the notes on copyright and usage.

Distribution, publication, and copying in any form are prohibited and subject to damages.

Table of contents

Introduction 9

#1 11

#2 16

#3 21

#4 25

#5 29

#6 34

#7 39

#8 43

#9 48

#10 53

Overview of All Titles in the Series "Ten Hypnoses" 58

Copying, publishing, and sharing with third parties are only permitted with the written consent of the author. Please observe the notes on copyright and usage.

Distribution, publication, and copying in any form are prohibited and subject to damages.

Copying, publishing, and sharing with third parties are only permitted with the written consent of the author. Please observe the notes on copyright and usage.

Introduction

The series "Ten Hypnoses" is very well known in Germany, Austria, and Switzerland as a collection of texts for therapeutic work and is used by numerous psychotherapeutic practices, doctors, therapists, coaches, and other helping professionals. I am pleased to now be able to offer these texts in other countries as well.

Most therapists have their own methods for inducing and deepening trance as well as for exiting trance. Therefore, I have focused on the main part of the hypnosis. The texts in this book can be integrated as the main part into any hypnosis process.

The texts in this collection use various hypnosis techniques. I will not explain these in detail, as I assume that users have the appropriate training. It is also not necessary to understand the exact structure or functioning of the different parts. The texts can simply be read aloud, and they will have their effect.

Decide for yourself which text best suits your client or patient at any given time. You can also combine passages from different texts. It is not about using all ten hypnoses in sequence. It is a selection of possibilities.

I want to emphasize that books cannot replace therapy. Psychotherapy or other therapeutic treatments involve much more. A careful diagnosis is the necessary basis for deciding on the use of methods, including whether hypnosis or one of my texts should be used. Even in this case, preparatory discussions, follow-up discussions during the session, and of course, a therapeutic concept for the sequence of sessions and the content approaches are essential parts of therapy. This cannot and should not be achieved with a collection of texts.

In any case, I wish you much success in your work and I am pleased if my text templates can contribute in a small way.

Ingo Michael Simon

#1

From now on, you will completely change your eating habits... ... You will eat more consciously and healthily for your body... ... This is the best decision you could have made because you now want to achieve and maintain a slim figure... ... It's truly amazing how well you can implement this decision today... ... to take the first big step today... ...

You can do it because it is your firm will to lose weight and become lighter... ... much lighter... ...

You will change your eating habits... ... You will take enough time for your meal... ... You will enjoy the sight of the food and first taste it with your eyes... ... This way, you let the food affect you... ... Then you can take in the smell, and you feel if you really have an appetite for what is in front of you... ... You feel whether you are really hungry... ... and if you are already full, you feel that you are full... ... or almost full... ...

And whenever you are full, you simply leave your meal... ... Whenever you are full, you simply leave your meal... ... because you are already full... ...

You take in the smell of the food intensely, and you can enjoy every bite... ... You chew your food slowly and for a long time... ... slowly and for a long time... ... You take your time... ... Eating slowly pays off for you... ... Eating slowly pays off for you... ...

As soon as your body has taken in enough, just as much as you need to feel good, your stomach closes immediately... ... Your stomach closes immediately... ... Isn't it amazing that from now on your body supports you in losing weight... ... to become slim and stay slim... ...

You take your time eating... ... This way, you lose more weight day by day until you reach your optimal and healthy weight for your body... ... You feel completely comfortable and are happy that your subconscious supports you so well... ...

And whenever you are full, you simply leave your meal... ... Whenever you are full, you simply leave your meal... ... Your stomach closes, and you leave the food... ...

You can easily forgo everything that makes you gain weight... ... Sweets and fatty foods are indifferent to you... ... You completely reject sweets... ... You completely reject sweets... ...

Your body naturally craves what is good and healthy for you and what supports you in losing weight... ... Your body knows what supports you in losing weight... ... And you only crave healthy foods... ... You lose weight day by day and week by week... ... until you reach your optimal and healthy weight... ... You become slimmer and feel better... ... You become slimmer and feel much better... ...

And whenever you are full, you simply leave your meal... ... Whenever you are full, you simply leave your meal... ...

Your pulse remains normal, your circulation is stable, and your body functions optimally... ... Your subconscious adjusts everything for you so that your metabolism and all your body functions work perfectly... ... You become slim and healthy... ... slim and healthy... ...

You are absolutely consistent. Sweets are indifferent to you... ... You reject sweets... ... You completely reject sweets... ... You completely reject sweets... ... You leave everything that unnecessarily makes you gain weight... ... You are absolutely consistent in this... ... You are absolutely consistent... ...

You now feel how the effect of my words spreads throughout your body. Your subconscious now sets everything optimally. It informs every single cell of your body... ... Every cell of your body now knows that you reject sweets... ... every cell of your body knows that you reject fatty foods, every cell knows that you only eat healthily... ...

And whenever you are full, you simply leave your meal... ... Whenever you are full, you simply leave your meal... ...

You take your time eating... ... This way, you lose more weight day by day until you reach your optimal and healthy weight for your body... ... You feel completely comfortable and are happy that your subconscious supports you so well... ...

As soon as your body has taken in enough, just as much as you need to feel good, your stomach closes immediately... ... Your stomach closes immediately... ... Isn't it amazing that from now on your body supports you in losing weight... ... to become slim and stay slim... ...

All these words are deeply embedded in your subconscious... ... Everything happens just as I have told you... ... Your subconscious will use tonight to embed all my words even deeper... ... as if you were dreaming a dream about eating less and becoming slimmer... ...

... ... Very deeply embedded is your will to lose weight... ... You feel better and healthier every day, slimmer and fitter... ... slimmer and fitter... ... Until you reach your optimal and healthy weight... ... And every morning when you look in the mirror, your body adjusts completely to feeling full quickly... ...

#2

You have decided to change your eating habits today... ... You are determined to eat more consciously and do something good for your body... ... This is the only decision you could make because only this way can you truly achieve your goal of becoming and staying slim... ... It is truly remarkable how well you can maintain this decision, to take a new path now... ... to take the decisive step into a slim and healthy future today... ... You can do it because it is your own will to lose weight and become lighter... ... much lighter... ...

You will change your eating habits... ... You decide to eat slowly... ... very slowly... ... and enjoy every bite thoroughly... ...You take your time for your meals... ... You first close your eyes at the table and take in the smell of the food intensely... ... This way, you let the food affect you with your eyes closed... ... Then you can take in the smell and feel if you really have an appetite for what is in front of you... ... You feel whether you are really hungry... ... and if you are already full, you feel that you are full... ... or almost full... ... You make it clear at every moment how much you really and actually want to take in... ... And whenever you are full, you simply leave your meal... ... Whenever you are full, you simply leave your meal... ... because you are already full... ... then you don't need any more food... ... You feel good even without food... ...

You take in the smell of the food intensely, and you can enjoy every bite... ... You chew your food slowly and for a long time... ... slowly and for a long time... ... You take your time... ... Eating slowly pays off for you... ... Eating slowly pays off for you... ... Eating slowly means enjoyment for you... ... and that's what you are: an enjoyer... ...

As soon as your body has taken in enough, just as much as you need to feel good, you stop eating immediately... ... You immediately feel that you are full... ... Isn't it amazing that from now on your body supports you in losing weight... ... to become slim and stay slim... ... And isn't it equally remarkable that your body can actually signal to you very clearly that you are already full... ...

You take your time eating... ... You enjoy every meal... ... because you eat slowly and with enjoyment... ... This way, you lose more weight day by day until you reach your optimal and healthy weight for your body... ... You feel completely comfortable and are happy that your subconscious supports you so well... ...

As soon as your body has taken in enough, just as much as you need to feel good, you stop eating immediately... ... You immediately feel that you are full... ... Isn't it amazing that from now on your body supports you in losing weight... ... to become slim and stay slim... ... And isn't it equally remarkable that your body can actually signal to you very clearly that you are already full... ...

Your body naturally craves what is good and healthy for you and what supports you in losing weight... ... Your body knows what supports you in losing weight... ... And you only crave healthy foods... ... You lose weight day by day and week by week... ... until you reach your optimal and healthy weight... ... You become slimmer and feel better... ... You become slimmer and feel much better... ...

As soon as your body has taken in enough, just as much as you need to feel good, you stop eating immediately... ... You immediately feel that you are full... ... Isn't it amazing that from now on your body supports you in losing weight... ... to become slim and stay slim... ... And isn't it equally remarkable that your body can actually signal to you very clearly that you are already full... ...

You are absolutely consistent. Sweets are indifferent to you... ... You reject sweets... ... You completely reject sweets... ... You completely reject sweets... ... As soon as you even think of sweets, you feel the craving for fresh fruit and vegetables... ... You leave everything that unnecessarily makes you gain weight... ... You are absolutely consistent in this... ... You are absolutely consistent... ... You now feel how the effect of your own decision spreads throughout your body. You completely adjust to feeling full again as soon as that is the case... ... You completely adjust to eating fruit and vegetables again... ... You completely adjust to rejecting sweets... ...

As soon as your body has taken in enough, just as much as you need to feel good, you stop eating immediately... ... You immediately feel that you are full... ... Isn't it amazing that from now on your body supports you in losing weight... ... to become slim and stay slim... ... And isn't it equally remarkable that your body can actually signal to you very clearly that you are already full... ...

Your subconscious completely adjusts to your new nutrition program... ... You can rely on your subconscious to help you... ... As soon as you sit down to eat, you immediately remember that you will only eat as much as you actually need... ... As soon as you sit down to eat, your body completely adjusts to informing you as soon as you are full... ... And you will immediately listen to this signal and stop eating... ...

#3

You want to lose weight... ... This goal is set, and you have already done a lot for it... ... Today, you can take a big and decisive step... ... You can set your subconscious to feel full faster today... ... You can also set your body to feel full faster... ... Both are directly connected... ... As soon as your body feels full, it can inform your subconscious that you should stop eating... ... that you also feel the fullness clearly in your thoughts and feelings... ... Your subconscious can also decide that you are full and inform your body to send the fullness signal clearly to you... ...

.. ... Today we are working with an anchor, we have already talked about it... ... You already carry this anchor on your body... ... your left hand is the anchor that is triggered by your right hand... ... But we will get to that a little later... ... To use the anchor one hundred percent, find the best position to trigger it now... ... Reach with your right hand to your left and feel for the ball of your hand with your fingers... ... very lightly... ... very gently... ... Decide whether you want to grasp the ball of your hand with your thumb and forefinger or with your thumb and middle finger... ... maybe you even have another variant... ... Do it the way you can best grasp the ball of your hand... ... [Wait until the client has found a good grip; encourage again if they do not join in immediately]... ... Wonderful... ... This works best... ... very good... ... And now let go of your hand again and place both hands loosely next to your body... ...

... ... Now it is time to find a very deep relaxation... ... deeper than ever before... ... You go deeper and deeper into yourself... ... as if you could sink into yourself... ... You let go of all thoughts... ... and you pay close attention to your body feeling... ... You feel how full you are at this moment... ... You are really full... ... Isn't it remarkable how easily you can feel this feeling so clearly?... ... As soon as you have made a decision, you can act... ... You make it completely clear at this moment that you have long made a decision... ... You have decided to eat less to lose weight... ... to take care of your health... ... to take good care of yourself... ... So you need no more than a single second to act on your decision... ... From now on, you simply do what is necessary to make your decision a reality... ... to feel that you are already full... ... just like now... ... Now, at this very moment, you can feel that you are full... ...

You feel the deep desire within you to feel this feeling every time you eat a normal portion... ... You imagine that you eat only one slice of bread with some cold cuts or cheese in the morning and evening, or with a topping that you particularly like, and are just as full as you are now... ... You imagine that you eat only one normally filled plate at noon or for your main meal and are just as full as you are now... ...

... ... You have decided, so you can act... ... In the word 'act' is the word 'hand'... ... Now you can actually act... ... Reach for your left hand... ... Do it now as you practiced... ... Grab your left hand and focus on your inner feeling of fullness... ... If you think the feeling of fullness should become even clearer, then just let it become even clearer and more intense in your feeling... ... even more intense... ... with even more mindfulness and care for yourself... ... just like that... ... just like that... ... You can do it... ...

... ... And now let this feeling become completely conscious... ... and now press the ball of your left hand... ...

and once again... ... press... ... Your inner self adjusts to the fact that exactly this pressing of the ball of the hand is the signal to immediately feel that you are truly full... ... Whenever you press the ball of your hand, you feel full and feel the need to take care of yourself... ... to take yourself seriously... ... to be important to yourself... ... Your body is relaxed and your hands are completely calm... ... Your body understands how your anchor works... ... It has already stored it for you so that you can use it again and again... ...

... ... Whenever you press the ball of your hand, you feel truly full and feel the need to take care of yourself... ... to take yourself seriously... ... to be important to yourself... ... It will soon become second nature for you to press or massage the ball of your hand, which works just like now... ... just like now... ... You have decided... ... You have acted... ...

#4

Losing weight is your goal... ... You have firmly resolved to finally become slim and stay slim... ... to eat only as much as you need to be full... ... and you can feel full much faster and more sustainably than you previously thought... ... and for you, it is the best decision you could make to eat less now and still be full... ...

... ... You have long wanted to eat less... ... to eat only three times a day... ... to eat less and be full... ... Now it should finally become true and remain true... ... You accomplish this today... ... Today we are working with an anchor, we have already talked about it... ... Maybe you are already wondering how quickly this anchor will work... ... how quickly the smell you will soon learn will help you lose weight... ... It may surprise you how well this anchor works... ... how quickly you actually feel full when you perceive the smell... ...

... ... Today is the first day of your new life... ... in a life where you manage to feel full after a normal portion... ... The good thing is that it is much easier than you previously thought... ... Even between meals, you can ensure that you simply feel full... ... Maybe you are wondering how you can feel full as quickly and as best as possible and feel good after a small portion of food... ...

... ... It is easier than you thought... ... You now feel the sensation of fullness... ... You are now full, and if you think this feeling should become even clearer, then just focus even more intensively on this beautiful and pleasant feeling... ... Relax even deeper and feel how full you are now... ...

Take a deep breath and feel how your chest expands... ... That's how good inner freedom feels... ... That's how good it feels to be full... ... just as full and satisfied as now... ... just as full and satisfied as now... ... And if you want, you feel even more clearly that you are really full... ... This is exactly the feeling you need between meals... ... This is exactly the feeling you need after a small portion of food... ... This is exactly the feeling you need every day... ...

... ... You can secure it... ... You can make sure that it also works in your waking everyday life... ... just like now... ... every day just like now... ... It is very simple... ... You can go into this feeling every day and feel good... ... You can decide every day when you want to be full... ...

... ... [Open the bottle with the aroma and move it towards the client's nose; hold it there]... ...

Take a deep breath and consciously perceive the smell you are experiencing... ... a pleasant smell... ... at the same time, you feel very clearly that you are actually full... ... Your good feeling and this smell you perceive now combine... ... They belong together... ... This smell and fullness belong closely together... ... This smell means: Yes, I am full!... ... Yes, I am full!... ...

... ... And whenever you smell this smell, you feel full... ... Whenever you perceive exactly this smell, you clearly feel that you are full... ... Even if you only think of the smell, you can already feel that you are becoming full... ... Your subconscious memorizes this smell and associates it with fullness... ...

... ... [Now close the bottle and put it away]... ...

... ... Continue breathing calmly and enjoy the peace... ... Give yourself mindfulness and attention and trust your subconscious to support you in quickly reaching this state again by simply smelling the bottle with the scent I just presented to you... ...

You can even test it... ... As soon as you perceive the smell, you feel full... ... It is as if you were having a small snack... ... Taking in this scent means becoming full... ...

... ... [Open the bottle again and hold it to the client's nose so they can clearly perceive the smell; hold it there briefly and then close it again]... ...

... ... It feels good... ... very, very good... ... Your inner self firmly embeds that even reaching for the bottle with your personal fullness scent triggers the signal in your body: Yes, I am full!... ... Yes, I am full!... ...

#5

You have realized that it is time to reconsider your eating habits and then change them... ... You have eaten too much in the past... ... You have now decided to lose weight... ... You have decided to become slim and stay slim... ... You want to change your eating habits... ... To do this, you set out on a journey into the past... ... You want to find out why you have been eating so much all these years... ... Today's journey can show you how it once started... ... At the same time, you find a new path today, because the past is gone... ... You can close it today... ...

... ... You imagine standing in front of a mirror and looking at yourself...

... First, take a look at yourself and assess what you want to change about your appearance... ... Take your time and look at yourself in peace... ... Let your own figure affect you... ... Also, look at your posture... ... Decide what you want to change... ... How should your figure look?... ... How should your posture be?... ... Take a moment and imagine how you want to look...

...... [Pause for about a minute, then continue]... ...

...... Now your journey should begin... ... your journey into the past... ... Time slowly runs backward... ... You look in the mirror and see yourself gradually getting younger... ... Meanwhile, your appearance changes... ...

...... You get younger as you go back in time... ... You want to find the time when you still ate normally... ... You want to find the time when you still had a normal weight... ... Over time, you will actually become thinner in the mirror... ... You may also get smaller because you started eating too much and gaining weight already in childhood... ... You get closer and closer to the time... ... You come closer and closer to the origin of your eating behavior... ... You even go back a little further, to a time when you were still slim, when you still ate normally... ... Finally, you reach the time when you still ate normally... ... You are now in that time and look around...

...... [Pause for about a minute, then continue]... ...

...... Look around and see where you are... ... Some things are different from today... ... You feel much freer and more comfortable in this earlier time... ... You have a completely different body feeling and a completely different mood in you... ... Immerse yourself deeply in this good feeling and let it work for you... ... This is how you once felt, and it was good... ... Let this good feeling become very intense again... ... This is how free you once felt... ... completely unburdened... ... completely light... ... and you were slim... ... inwardly light and outwardly light... ... Immerse yourself completely in this good feeling... ... Let the feeling of being slim and light become very clear... ... even clearer... ...

... ... This feeling helps you to become as slim as you were back then... ... exactly as free as back then... ... exactly as light... ...

You anchor the good feeling deeply within you... ... You imprint it firmly and hold it inwardly... ... You take it with you on your journey through time... ... You take the good feeling from back then with you and can always carry it with you... ...

... ... Then time slowly runs forward again, and you come to the time when something changed... ... You reach the time when you started eating too much... ... You look around here too... ... You have taken the good feeling from the time before with you... ... So you also feel comfortable and satisfied now... ... Like an observer in this past time, you can calmly get a picture of how it once was... ... You understand why you started eating so much... ... At the same time, you feel that you no longer need this... ... Back then, it had to happen, but not today... ... With the good feeling of the earlier slim time in your luggage, you can now stay calm and composed... ... You can now say goodbye to the idea of eating a lot... ... It belongs to this long-forgotten time... ...

... ... It is like saying goodbye to an old friend... ... It can also be difficult, but it is possible because you carry the strength of the slim time deep within you... ... and because you know that the idea of eating a lot comes from the past and is no longer needed today... ... You leave the idea of eating a lot exactly there... ... It stays in the past, where it belongs... ... But you let time continue to move forward and slowly approach your present day again... ... With a good mood in your luggage, you slowly approach today's day... ... The idea of eating a lot stays in the past... ... That is where it belongs...

... ... You see your reflection... ... You see yourself getting older again and arriving in the present... ... But your reflection is slim... ... You have become light inwardly, and therefore you also see your slim reflection... ... The more you think about the idea of eating a lot belonging to the past, the slimmer your image becomes... ... You feel that you are full and need much less food than before... ...

... ... You set yourself inwardly to eat less because you no longer need the much food... ... You sharpen your sense of when you are truly hungry... ... You first check every feeling of appetite... ... You consider whether it comes from past needs and then send it to the past... ... Your sense for the present becomes stronger and stronger, and you can recognize when you are truly hungry... ...

#6

Today, you can find answers to a question that is particularly close to your heart... ... You have often asked yourself this question: Why did I become so overweight?... ... Many reasons may have occurred to you... ... you may have already found some answers... ... But then there was always the feeling that something was missing... ... something you should still see and understand... ... so that you can completely free yourself from this old pattern... ... so that from today on, you can set yourself even more and more intensely to eat in a way that makes you slim and keeps you slim... ... You are determined to find these answers and recognize today what made you eat so much that you became so overweight... ... You will also find the function that being overweight had for you... ... because somewhere there is also a positive function that you no longer need... ...

... ... So you fully prepare for deep relaxation... ... You feel the peace and relaxation at this moment, and it can go even deeper... ... Follow your breathing with mindfulness and feel the rhythm of your breath... ...

Imagine a beautiful and very pleasant place... ... a place where you can feel very comfortable... ... maybe there is such a favorite place because you have been there often... ... or there is such a place in your imagination... ... somewhere in nature or by the sea... ... possibly simply surrounded by light and warmth... ... as an inner place in a beautiful feeling... ...

... ... Then you can imagine that your own memories and feelings are like balloons that slowly rise up... ... slowly float into the sky as if they were filled with gas... ... Balloons of your own feelings... ...

First, some balloons rise that carry the burdens of the past week... ... But now the balloons are light and rise into the sky... ... feather-light... ... The balloons take all your burdens with them... ... so it can become even calmer inside you and much lighter... ... So you can now simply let go of the burdens and stress of the past week... ... The balloons free you from them and rise lightly into the sky... ... You can watch them... ... You can watch your burdens fade away...

... At the same time, you feel the inner relief and feel lighter... ... lighter inside... ... lighter in your feelings... ... The lighter you feel inside, the lighter your body can become... ... This is an important step... ... Watch the balloons... ... The more clearly you imagine the balloons, the more burdens actually dissolve... ... Just watch them... ... exactly like that... ... That's right... ...

... ... Then a large, very thick balloon slowly rises... ... It is a very special balloon that rises... ... It knows why you accumulated this overweight... ... This balloon knows what special function the overweight had... ... back when it started... ... and maybe there is still a trace of this function today... ... The balloon rises before your inner eye, and you can read a word on its surface that shows you what your overweight was for... ... Look at it and observe the balloon... ... You can recognize the word... ...

... ... Maybe it says protection because your body mass was supposed to be a kind of protective shield... ... Maybe it says distance because you wanted or even had to keep other people away from you... ... maybe certain people or even a specific person... ... But maybe there is a completely different word on your balloon... ... Let it become clearer, whatever you can recognize on your balloon... ... It shows you what your overweight was for... ... Let the word just affect you...

... ... [Pause for about a minute, then continue]... ...

... ... Let the balloon rise higher and higher until you can no longer see it... ... In doing so, make it clear to yourself that you no longer need this function of your overweight... ... Maybe the overweight still seemingly serves you because the circumstances that led to you needing it are still partly there... ... and yet... ... You have become much stronger over the years... ... You have built up strength and resilience... ... You can also deal with yourself and your environment in other ways... ... You know that today you can protect yourself better than back then... ...

... ... Then suddenly many balloons rise... ... hundreds of colorful balloons rise and fly into the sky... ... Inside you, so many anxieties and entanglements dissolve that now hundreds of balloons rise, and you become lighter and lighter... ...

... ... Now you know what your overweight was once for... ... At the same time, you know more clearly than ever that you no longer need this function... ... You can handle it differently, you can take care of yourself even if you are slim... ... You can do it... ... Now it is time to be light inside... ... and light outside... ... Now it is truly and actually time to be light inside... ... and light outside...

... ... Your inner self firmly imprints that you can now be slim... ... and whenever you see an inflated balloon, you feel very clearly that now is the time when you can be light and slim... ... Then, all by itself, your eating habits will change, and you will become lighter... ... Every morning, you already look at the balloon... ... before every meal, you look at the balloon, and immediately you feel how full it actually makes you...

... ... [Discuss with your client that they should inflate a balloon and write the found word on it. They should look at it in the morning after getting up and preferably before every meal. So, an "anchor" is additionally available.]...

#7

Hold the client's arm at the wrist and pull it diagonally upwards without overstretching the arm. Test during the holding suggestion by slightly giving way to see if the arm is already cataleptic and let go as soon as the catalepsy stands.

You want to lose weight and know that some changes are required... ... You want to give up sweets from now on... ... You know that it is easiest if you manage to neutralize sweets... ... make them unimportant so that you could eat them but don't have to... ... so that you can simply leave them lying or even reject them because they no longer matter... ... Maybe you are wondering how that works, neutralizing sweets... ... You know it's possible, otherwise, you wouldn't be here today to neutralize sweets... ... Today, I will show you how to do it... ... You yourself can do it deep inside... ... your inner self can do it... ... and it can also show you as soon as it has done it... ... For this, we use your arm... ... because your inner self... ... your subconscious can show you with your arm as soon as sweets are neutralized...

… [Now, the client's arm is held by the therapist until the catalepsy stands. Discuss the procedure with the client before the session and always announce touches during the trance immediately. Always avoid startle or defensive reactions!] …

… … I now take your wrist and hold your arm for you… … Just allow it… … Everything happens for your well-being…

… [Now hold the client's arm at the wrist and pull it diagonally upwards without overstretching the arm. Test during the subsequent holding suggestion by slightly giving way to see if the arm is already cataleptic and let go as soon as the catalepsy stands.] …

… … Now focus on your arm. It becomes firmer and firmer, as firm as an iron bar… and feather-light… so it is very easy to hold the arm… to hold it up as if it were held by an invisible balloon… Your arm becomes firmer and firmer… firmer and firmer, very firm and stable… Your arm takes on posture and remains in exactly this position… Your arm becomes stiff and firm and stays in exactly this position… It is light and very firm… Your arm is completely immovable and stiff... completely immovable and stiff... Your arm remains in exactly this position... just like that...

... [If necessary, extend a bit more if the arm is not held, which should happen quickly. For the client, the cataleptic state is not a subjective burden or strain. They have the feeling that the arm holds itself.] ...

Now I give your subconscious the task to neutralize sweets... They become meaningless to you... You will no longer feel a desire for sweets... on the contrary... You will even reject them because they no longer taste good... Your subconscious now adjusts to neutralize sweets... Your arm shows you how much your subconscious has already achieved...

Your arm will now slowly become movable again and slowly sink to the support... This happens in exactly the time your subconscious needs to completely neutralize sweets so that you no longer need them and can reject them... Your arm now becomes movable and sinks downwards, and as soon as the arm touches the support, all sweets have become completely meaningless to you... As soon as your arm touches the support, you feel freed from all sweets...

You no longer want them because they no longer taste good...

... [Wait until the arm sinks onto the support. This may take some time but can also happen quickly. The speed does not matter for success. It is an indication of how strong the will to change is and how big any doubts are. Just let the process run as it happens. If the arm does not move, help with the following or similar suggestions.]

Take your time... ... Do it at your speed... ... in your tempo... ... As soon as the right time is there, your arm will also move... ...

Surely today is the right day for it, then your arm will also move soon... ...

If today is not yet the right day, then your arm will not move today, but if today is the right day, it will move soon... ...

You are now completely free from sweets... ... completely free... ... Sweets are now completely meaningless to you... ...

#8

to deal with your old thinking patterns and everything that led to your overweight... ... Everything that is deep in our soul is also found in our body... ... Every thought, every mood... ... every single feeling is reflected in our body... ... shows up there as pressure... ... as tension... ... as a strange feeling... ... sometimes even as pain... ... or just as a strange tingling... ... So if you can clearly feel your body, you can also achieve everything you have set out to do... ... understand everything... ... and change everything... ...

... ... Somewhere in your body, the old thinking patterns that led to your weight accumulation also sit... ... Let's call it your overweight pattern... ... It sits deep inside you and works from there without you noticing it... ... But by now you know it... ... You have long understood that there must be this special pattern... ... You have accepted that it is there... ... At the same time, you have set out to find and dissolve it... ...

... ... It is anchored in your feelings and thoughts, but also in your body... ... You can feel it in your body... ... Maybe you know that you can feel everything that belongs to you physically when you come to rest, as you are now... ... and concentrate on your body... ... as you are now... ... Of course, you have experienced in your everyday life how your overweight pattern can manifest, but it also shows up in your body... ... just differently... ... as tension... ... as warmth or cold... ... as pressure or in another way... ... All thinking patterns that we carry deep inside us show up most clearly at a specific point in our body... ... as a signal that we can perceive... ... So a signal of your overweight pattern also shows up in your body, warning you... ... so that you do not fall into the trap of overeating again... ... so that you can take better care of yourself... ... You just need to recognize this spot, then you can work on it and build a new pattern... ...

... ... Now focus on your body and feel your body... ... Scan down from head to toe, like a scanner, and find this special spot... ... Find this spot that feels different because your overweight pattern sits there... ... You find it... ... It feels different... ... maybe just a bit colder or warmer... ... maybe as a tingling... ... or as a slight goosebump that suddenly forms... ... Wherever this spot is... ... Your overweight pattern shows up there through a physical signal... ... right there... ... But even if you haven't found it... ... It is there... ... Then just take the spot that comes to your mind spontaneously... ... wherever that is... ...

... ... Feel deeper and deeper into it... ... Go right into this feeling... ... whatever it may be... ... It is your overweight that you feel there... ... Go deeper and deeper into this spot in your body and feel the signals of your body more clearly... ... Maybe it feels strenuous or burdensome... ... Maybe you thought you had already overcome it more... ... Do not worry, because here you mainly feel the thinking pattern that led to your body fullness... ...

... ... Now direct all your attention and all your mindfulness and loving care to exactly this point in your body and connect with the inner pattern that lies there... ... Imagine a warm feeling radiating from this spot in all directions... ... as if an inner sun at exactly this spot spreads its light and warmth gently in all directions... ... Let it get warmer and warmer, as pleasant as possible... ... Imagine bright light radiating from this spot into the depths of your body... ... and also outward... ... Let this spot in your body become a source of warmth and become more and more pleasant for you... ... This warmth can capture your whole body because you bring this mindfulness... ... this attention to yourself... ... So this spot in your body becomes calmer... ... more relaxed... ... more pleasant... ... and just as pleasantly, the thinking pattern changes... ... More and more old entanglements dissolve and are replaced by new patterns of self-care and mindfulness... ... Everywhere, where recently the overweight pattern was, you find more and more love from you for yourself... ... more and more love from you for yourself... ... your self-love and mindfulness... ... your self-love and mindfulness... ... Keep breathing calmly and evenly and trust the power within you... ... Everywhere, where recently the overweight pattern was, you find more and more love from you for yourself... ... more and more love from you for yourself... ... your self-love and mindfulness... ... your self-love and mindfulness...

... ... You feel the change in your body and make it clear to yourself that your body can always show you how you feel in your feelings... ... especially in the feelings that you couldn't always feel so well in everyday life... ... Now you can, because you know that your body helps you... ... So every day, you pay attention to your body and ask yourself already in the morning when you get up how your body feels today... ... It shows you what you need to pay attention to... ... Whenever you find a spot that feels noticeably different from the rest of your body, you give yourself mindfulness and focus on this spot... ... In doing so, you connect with the feeling that lies within you and recognize it... ... So you can react... ... So you can recognize in time when you need to take better care of yourself...

#9

You go into the land of dreams... ... You stand in the middle of a meadow, and the weather is beautiful... ... The sun is shining and invites you to hike over the four high mountains... ... You see them in front of you... four mountains of challenge... You have often faced great challenges... Many you managed well... others were more difficult... Maybe you couldn't handle some tasks or not as you expected from yourself... And today is about the special challenge of becoming lighter and slimmer... today and every day of your life, because you want to be slim forever... So you set off... you carry a backpack with four meals with you, so you are always full on the way... So go ahead into your slimmer future... Step by step, you will become lighter on your hike in this beautiful fantasy and then every day in your waking reality... lighter every day...Your path leads to the first mountain... It is the mountain of longing... All unfulfilled wishes are here to be found and all dreams of a better time... You remember your longings and wishes... everything unfulfilled... You think about what you have not yet been able to achieve... and what you wish for your future... You go further and further up the mountain of longing... Up here, you can see infinitely far into the distance... You know that you have often eaten something to numb longings... So you could give yourself something that was denied to you elsewhere... If you are lighter... as light as now here in this beautiful daydream where you can hike without getting tired... then it is much easier to climb the mountain of longing and feel which unfulfilled wishes you still have... At the summit cross of this mountain, you say to yourself: Eating is the wrong way... I simply fulfill my real wishes... You open your backpack and leave a meal at the summit cross and leave it there... You don't need it anymore... You have enough other goals... You can eat later... And then you go down into the valley and become lighter... You have overcome a hurdle and come closer and closer to yourself and your real needs... Your path leads you further... and with ease, you reach the second mountain... It is the mountain of perfectionism... You climb up and think about what role perfectionism has played in your life so far... You have often tried to be perfect... maybe also to think and feel perfectly... to fulfill something even though you had completely different interests... And although your eating habits are not exactly perfect, you probably have the excessive demand to be completely disciplined now... There is again the demand for perfectionism... You climb higher and higher... You make it clear to yourself that it was sometimes the unfulfilled perfectionism that made you eat... As if you wanted to fill something... At the summit cross of this mountain, you say to yourself: Eating is the wrong way... I don't have to be perfect... I am good as I am... You open your backpack and leave a meal at the summit cross and leave it there... You don't need it anymore... You have enough other goals... You can eat later... And then you go down into the valley and become lighter...Your path leads further to the third mountain... It is the mountain of guilt... ... You know that well... So often, you had a guilty conscience because you thought you were doing something wrong or not fulfilling something... Even when you thought entirely about yourself, it felt like selfishness, and you had a guilty conscience... Of course, also when eating... When you then ate far too much, you often got annoyed afterward and had a guilty conscience... So you also climb this mountain of challenge and think about the situations where you often had a guilty conscience... Many situations that were always associated with a guilty conscience come to mind... Some may be deeply hidden, but you can at least develop a feeling for them... At the summit cross of this mountain, you say to yourself: Eating is the wrong way... I let go of the guilt and become light... You open the backpack and leave a meal at the summit cross and leave it there... You don't need it anymore... You have enough other goals... You can eat later... And then you go down into the valley and become lighter... Your path leads you further and brings you to the fourth mountain... It is the mountain of lightness... Your backpack has already become much lighter because you have left something to eat on every mountain... You don't need it anymore... Now you climb the mountain of lightness, and with every step, you become lighter and fuller... Because both go together... being full and being light... being full and being light... On the way up, you think about the last time you felt inwardly light... You think about the situations and occasions when you can feel light... You think about what you need today or tomorrow to be light... light and relaxed and at the same time satisfied... You climb higher and higher on this mountain and take the feeling of lightness deep inside you... Lightheartedness and cheerfulness... deep inside you... Liberation deep inside you... And all that makes you full and satisfied... At the summit cross of this mountain, you say to yourself: Eating is the wrong way... I allow myself lightness and freedom... You open your backpack and leave a meal at the summit cross and leave it there... You don't need it anymore... You have enough other goals... You can eat later... And then you go down into the valley and become lighter... Your backpack is empty... You have left all meals and feel free... In the valley, you continue to wander and collect lots of green clovers... Each clover stands for a beautiful daydream and for a new idea... for an enrichment of your life... for new goals and the feeling of freedom that can be associated with it... You enjoy the day and are free...

... ... Then you think that maybe it's not only like this in the land of dreams but also in your everyday life... ... Fantasy and reality are much closer together than you thought... ... You think about how the land of dreams is deep inside you. It has always been there. I am just telling you about it... ...

#10

You go into the land of dreams... ... You stand on a wide path and follow it quite naturally because you know it brings you closer to yourself... ... closer to your inner truth... ... but especially to parts of this truth that you do not yet know... ... Parts that you may have deliberately ignored for a long time... ...

... ... You just go full of trust and know that here in the land of dreams, you can always only find yourself... ... So you are protected and safe here... ... You follow the path into the valley... ... go deeper and deeper... ... very deep into the land of dreams... ... It becomes quieter and quieter... ... You arrive in the valley of silence... ... this valley where time seems to stand still... ... Here only the moment counts... ... only the immediate present... ... Even the last second belongs to the past and cannot be changed... ... Only the present can you shape and thus determine the future yourself... ... But you can learn from the past... ... You can see what you once did... ... what you couldn't change or even influence at the time... ... to now shape the present so that you can reach your goal better and faster... ... your goal of losing weight and finally being light... ...

... ... You finally arrive at the end of the valley and find a narrow path leading upward... ... You follow this path, and every step here in the land of dreams is feather-light... ... You keep going up... ... until you stand in the sun and can look far over the land... ... Your gaze goes far into the distance and is clearer than ever before... ...

... ... Then you come to a beautiful garden... ... From afar, you already see the colorful splendor... ... The gate opens by itself and lets you in... ... This is the garden of time... ... You follow this path further, which leads right through the garden of time... ... Then you come to a stone well... ... It is surrounded by beautiful plants... ... A place that invites you to linger... ...

... ... You go very close to the well and look into it... ... It is filled to the brim with clear water... ... But you cannot see the bottom because the well is infinitely deep... ... the well of truth... ... It exists only here in the land of your dreams and memories... ... the well of truth... ...

... ... You look at the water and see images rising from the depths of the well... ... They rise in the water and come to the surface... ... Pictures rise to the water's surface... ...

... ... Now a picture rises that shows you people who contributed to you deciding to become overweight at one point... ... You see them as if in a photo, like a poster rising from the depths and remaining on the water's surface to be seen by you... ... You look at the photo... ... Maybe you expected these very people because you always suspected that in contact with them, you made the decision to become overweight without noticing it at the time... ... You couldn't prevent it either... ... It happened as it did back then... ... But today, everything can be different... ... Today, you can learn from exactly this image to make a different decision... ... because today everything is already different... ... The image belongs to the past... ... But you can learn... ...

But maybe you also see people in this picture whom you did not expect... ... It can also be people you love and appreciate... ... But in contact with the very people you see, you once learned that it was better to be overweight... ... Maybe it is even just one single person you can see... ... the person who most or most clearly impressed you... ... Today, you can learn from exactly this person how to be light again... ... light inside and light outside... ...

... ... Then the image slowly dissolves... ... It dissolves on the surface because you have already understood everything and learned everything you need to successfully lose weight now... ... Look at the image and watch it dissolve... ...

... ... [Pause for about a minute, then continue]... ...

... ... Now breathe deeply... ... deeply in and out... ... deeply in and out... ... and feel the inner liberation... ... You may now feel light and become light... ...

... ... Then look at the sky and imagine how it will be when you have reached your desired weight... ... Now nothing can stop you... ... Now you are free from old constraints... ... Now you can lose weight and be slim... ... Imagine very clearly how beautiful it will be when you have completely succeeded in reaching your desired weight...

... ... Then you find a nice place near the well and lie down... ... You close your eyes and enjoy this beautiful light feeling inside you... ... You give yourself peace and mindfulness...

... ... Then you think that maybe it's not only like this in the land of dreams but also in your everyday life... ... Fantasy and reality are much closer together than you thought... ... You think about how the land of dreams is deep inside you. It has always been there. I am just telling you about it... ...

Overview of All Titles in the Series "Ten Hypnoses"

Volume 1: Smoking Cessation
Volume 2: Anxiety and Restlessness
Volume 3: Burnout
Volume 4: Reducing Overweight
Volume 5: Coping with the Past
Volume 6: Suicidal Thoughts and Attempts
Volume 7: Psycho-Oncology
Volume 8: Obsessions and Tics
Volume 9: Self-Confidence and Decision-Making
Volume 10: Grief Work
Volume 11: Psychosomatics
Volume 12: Chronic Pain
Volume 13: Depressive Thoughts
Volume 14: Panic Attacks
Volume 15: Domestic Violence, Victim Support
Volume 16: Post-Traumatic Stress
Volume 17: Exam Anxiety and Stage Fright
Volume 18: Anti-Violence Training, Offender Support
Volume 19: Addiction Tendencies
Volume 20: Social Phobia and Fear of Contact
Volume 21: Nail Biting
Volume 22: Self-Awareness and Self-Love
Volume 23: Teeth Grinding and Night Clenching
Volume 24: Feelings of Guilt
Volume 25: Fear in Crowds
Volume 26: Fear of Flying, Aviophobia
Volume 27: Fear in Enclosed Spaces, Claustrophobia
Volume 28: Tinnitus, Ear Noises
Volume 29: Fear of Heights
Volume 30: Neurodermatitis

Volume 31: Finding Inner Balance
Volume 32: Overcoming Loneliness
Volume 33: Fear of Illness, Hypochondria
Volume 34: Anticipatory Anxiety, Fear of Fear
Volume 35: Jealousy in Relationships
Volume 36: Driving Anxiety
Volume 37: New Start after Separation
Volume 38: Fear of Injections
Volume 39: Heart Anxiety Neurosis
Volume 40: Overcoming Resentment and Anger
Volume 41: Resolving Blockages and Positive Thinking
Volume 42: Stress Reduction, Stress Management
Volume 43: Body Relaxation
Volume 44: Deep Relaxation
Volume 45: Fear of the Dark
Volume 46: Falling Asleep and Staying Asleep
Volume 47: Compulsive Buying
Volume 48: Restless Legs Syndrome
Volume 49: Bulimia
Volume 50: Anorexia
Volume 51: Overcoming Nightmares
Volume 52: Imagined Deformity
Volume 53: Overcoming Distrust, Finding Trust
Volume 54: Processing Failures
Volume 55: Humiliation, Emotional Hurt
Volume 56: Distressing Compassion, Vicarious Suffering
Volume 57: Self-Forgiveness
Volume 58: Self-Awareness, Self-Confidence
Volume 59: Saying No
Volume 60: Assertiveness
Volume 61: Setting Boundaries and Self-Assertion
Volume 62: Decision-Making Ability

- Volume 63: Success Orientation
- Volume 64: Ruminating, Circular Thinking
- Volume 65: Accepting Pregnancy
- Volume 66: Birth Preparation
- Volume 67: Spiritual Opening
- Volume 68: Joy of Life and Inner Lightness
- Volume 69: Patience and Inner Peace
- Volume 70: Fibromyalgia and Rheumatism
- Volume 71: Irritable Bowel Syndrome, Crohn's Disease
- Volume 72: Fear of Nausea, Emetophobia
- Volume 73: Stuttering and Cluttering, Speech Flow Disorders
- Volume 74: Concentration and Knowledge Anchoring
- Volume 75: Vitality and Spontaneity
- Volume 76: Searching for Meaning and Finding Goals
- Volume 77: Life Crises, Life Events
- Volume 78: Workaholism, Goal Obsession
- Volume 79: Helper Syndrome, Helpless Helpers
- Volume 80: Medication Abuse
- Volume 81: Gambling Addiction
- Volume 82: Internet Addiction, Smartphone Addiction
- Volume 83: Hoarding Disorder, Compulsive Collecting
- Volume 84: Conspiracy Thoughts, Overvalued Ideas
- Volume 85: Fear of Operations and Treatments
- Volume 86: Fear of Aging
- Volume 87: Travel Anxiety
- Volume 88: Anxiety When Urinating, Paruresis
- Volume 89: Fear of Intimacy and Togetherness
- Volume 90: Fear of Blushing
- Volume 91: Coming Out in Homosexuality
- Volume 92: Charisma Training
- Volume 93: Migraines and Chronic Headaches
- Volume 94: Overcoming Allergies, Bronchial Asthma

Volume 95: Normalizing Blood Pressure
Volume 96: Compulsive Perfectionism
Volume 97: Sports Hypnosis, Motivation
Volume 98: Sports Hypnosis, Performance Enhancement
Volume 99: Determination and Focus
Volume 100: Encountering the Inner Child
Volume 101: Cravings, Binge Eating
Volume 102: Stimulating Metabolism
Volume 103: Bipolar Mood Swings
Volume 104: Borderline, Identity Crises
Volume 105: Hypomania, Euphoria, Mania
Volume 106: Restlessness, Agitation
Volume 107: Nervous Breakdown
Volume 108: Adjustment Disorders
Volume 109: Self-Alienation, Depersonalization
Volume 110: Ending Self-Pity
Volume 111: Primary Gain of Illness
Volume 112: Secondary Gain of Illness
Volume 113: Bullying, Victim Support
Volume 114: Letting Go of Envy and Jealousy
Volume 115: Fear of Spiders, Arachnophobia
Volume 116: Fear of Dogs or Cats
Volume 117: Fear of Strangers, Xenophobia
Volume 118: Excessive Worries, Generalized Anxiety
Volume 119: Strengthening Sense of Responsibility
Volume 120: Unrequited Love, Heartache
Volume 121: Work-Life Balance
Volume 122: Letting Go of Unattainable Goals
Volume 123: Allowing and Accepting Help
Volume 124: Letting Go of Adult Children
Volume 125: Tourette Syndrome
Volume 126: Life Changes and New Starts

Volume 127: Accepting Life in a Wheelchair
Volume 128: Understanding and Overcoming Homesickness
Volume 129: Understanding and Overcoming Wanderlust
Volume 130: Dizziness, Meniere's Disease
Volume 131: Overcoming Aggression
Volume 132: Cutting and Self-Harm
Volume 133: Hair Pulling, Trichotillomania
Volume 134: Postpartum Depression
Volume 135: For Relatives of Dementia Patients
Volume 136: Self-Harm, Artificial Disorders
Volume 137: Activating Self-Healing Powers
Volume 138: Preventing Depression Relapse
Volume 139: Reactive Psychoses, Follow-Up
Volume 140: Obsessive Thoughts and Impulses
Volume 141: Compulsive Checking
Volume 142: Compulsive Counting, Symmetry Obsession
Volume 143: Compulsive Washing, Cleanliness Obsession
Volume 144: Compulsive Questioning
Volume 145: Dissociative Paralysis
Volume 146: Phantom Pain
Volume 147: Overcoming Complaining
Volume 148: Hay Fever, Pollen Allergy
Volume 149: Sexual Abuse, Victim Support
Volume 150: Standing Strong Against Sexism, #metoo
Volume 151: Binge Eating
Volume 152: Overcoming Thoughts of Revenge
Volume 153: Detachment from the Aggressor, Stockholm Syndrome
Volume 154: Courage to Separate
Volume 155: Chronic Fatigue, Exhaustion
Volume 156: Fear of the Future, Existential Anxiety
Volume 157: Excessive Worry About Children
Volume 158: Fear of Failure

Volume 159: Ending Distrust and Control
Volume 160: Dejection, Dysphoria
Volume 161: Boreout, Chronic Boredom
Volume 162: Bipolar Disorders, Relapse Prevention
Volume 163: Mania, Relapse Prevention
Volume 164: Nihilism, Feelings of Worthlessness
Volume 165: Thumb Sucking
Volume 166: Being Brave
Volume 167: Being Proud
Volume 168: Overcoming Shyness
Volume 169: Being Able to Delegate Responsibility
Volume 170: Being Able to Show Emotions
Volume 171: Letting Go of Guilt, Victim Support
Volume 172: Processing Guilt, Offender Support
Volume 173: Mood Swings, Cyclothymia
Volume 174: Lack of Drive, Vital Sadness
Volume 175: Hearing Voices with Reality Reference
Volume 176: Confident Communication
Volume 177: Standing Up for Oneself
Volume 178: Taking New Paths
Volume 179: Confident Job Application
Volume 180: No Longer Being Taken Advantage Of
Volume 181: End of Submissiveness
Volume 182: Depressive Numbness
Volume 183: Mood Drops, Affective Incontinence
Volume 184: Mood Instability
Volume 185: Somatoform Disorders
Volume 186: Stomach Ulcer, Psychosomatic
Volume 187: Accepting Amputation
Volume 188: Overcoming and Letting Go of Hatred
Volume 189: Ending Accusations
Volume 190: Allowing Tears, Being Able to Cry

Volume 191: Finding and Sorting Repressed Feelings
Volume 192: Somatoform Pain
Volume 193: Living Autonomously
Volume 194: Anhedonia, Joylessness
Volume 195: Persistent Sadness
Volume 196: Obesity, Food Addiction
Volume 197: Parents of Abused Children
Volume 198: Letting Go and Letting Be
Volume 199: Childhood Sexual Abuse
Volume 200: Fear of Loss

www.ingramcontent.com/pod-product-compliance
Lightning Source LLC
Chambersburg PA
CBHW030504220526
45464CB00006B/2657